Lean And Green Mastery

An All-Inclusive Walkthrough Of Easy And Yummy Recipes To Eat Well Everyday And Lose Weight Fast Without Feeling On A Diet And Discover The Secrets Of The "Fuelings Hacks Meal

Lisa G. Torres

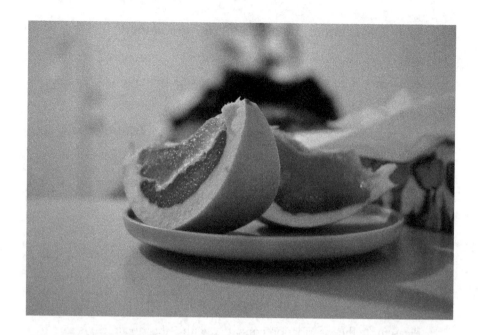

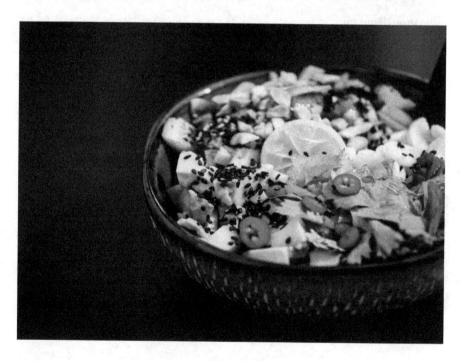

Table of Contents

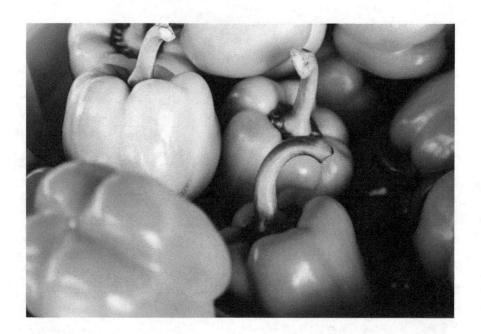

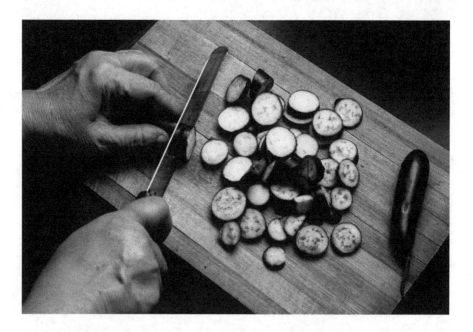

Introduction

I f you are looking to lose weight fast and you don't always have enough time to cook, this regimen is the best option for you. However, this diet program requires that you work with a coach on a one-on-one guide and counseling. It includes branded products known as Fuelings and homemade food known as Lean & Green meals.

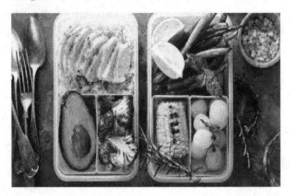

These Fuelings have over 60 products that are low in carb and high in protein. They have probiotic cultures with health-promoting bacteria that boost gut health. Some of them are bars, shakes, cereals, cookies, pasta, puddings, etc.

The Diet Programs

The program has three versions, which include 2 weight loss plans and a maintenance plan.

- **Optimal Weight 5&1**: This plan is the most popular among the program plans. It is made up of daily 5 Fuelings and 1 lean and green meal.

- **Optimal Weight 4&2&1**: If you need more calories, this plan is for you. It is more flexible and includes 4 Fuelings, 2 lean and green, and 1 snack every day.

- **Optimal Health 3&3**: With 3 Fuelings and 3 lean and green meals, it is designed to help in weight maintenance.

Diet Guide

For a quick weight loss goal, the Optimal Weight 5&1 Plan may be the best plan to start with. Most people with the target of losing weight usually go for this plan as it helps them to drop up to 12 pounds within 12 weeks.

In the Optimal Weight 5&1 Plan, you are expected to eat one lean and green meal and five Fuelings. These meals are to be eaten every 2-3 hours intervals. Then, you will back it up with 30 minutes of exercise. Your coach will direct you on the best approach.

However, the daily carbs from meals and Fuelings should not exceed 100 grams. You can get meals and Fuelings from the company. Though it may not be cost-effective, this book is designed to help you save costs. You can prepare the meals by yourself to reduce costs.

There are a plethora of recipes in this book to help you along the process for your daily meals. You can also eat out, but keep in mind that you must follow the diet plan as instructed by your coach. However, alcohol is highly restricted for this plan.

Once you get to your desired weight, you are expected to enter the maintenance phase. This is a transition phase that requires a gradual increase in your daily calorie intake to no more than 1,550 cal. You can add a wider variety of food to your daily meals, which include fruits, whole grains, and low-fat dairy.

The maintenance phase is expected to last for 6 weeks before you move to the Optimal Health 3&3 Plan. In this plan, your daily food intake will be 3 Fuelings and 3 lean and green meals.

In this diet, most people that follow the diet usually opt for the 5&1 plan. The 5&1 program is made up of 5 Fuelings and 1 high protein low-carb meal. There are over 60 fueling options in this diet, and these options include bars, puddings, shakes, soups, biscuits, etc. These Fuelings contain probiotics that help to promote digestive health.

The interesting aspect of this diet is its flexibility, which makes it easier to work with. Once you reach your desired weight goal, you can easily switch to the 3&3 plan. Transitioning to this weight-maintenance plan is easy since you have already changed the old unhealthy eating habits. For those looking to consume more calories, the 4&2&1 plan is your best bet. With the 4&2&1 plan, you take 4 Fuelings, 2 healthy lean and green meals, and 1 snack.

How This Diet Can Help You Lose Weight

How much weight you lose on the this diet depends mostly on how active and how you follow the plan. If you stick with the plan and stay very active, you will lose more weight. Many have tried it, and it worked perfectly well. The following research studies show how effective the diet can be when strictly followed. Though the research is mostly on Medifast, this diet and Medifast have identical macro-nutrients and can be interchanged to achieve the same result. So, the studies are valid for both this diet and Medifast plans.

- A study published in the Obesity journal in 2016 showed that after 12 weeks of observing the diet guides, obese people lost 8.8% body weight.

- The study released by John Hopkins Medicine that ran for 12 weeks revealed that weight-loss programs like Medifast are effective for a long-term weight loss goal.

- A study in the Nutrition Journal carried out in 2015 shows that 310 obese and overweight people who followed the diet plans lost 24 lb in 12 weeks. In the 24th week, the average weight loss recorded was 35 lb.

- Another study published in the Nutrition Journal shows that 90 obese adults who followed the 5&1 plan lost an average of 30 pounds in 16 weeks.

- The analysis published in the Eating and Weight Disorder Journal in 2008 shows that the average weight loss recorded on

324 obese patients in 12 weeks was 21 lb and 26 ½ lb after 24 weeks. However, these patients also took appetite suppressant.

Is Diet Easy To Follow?

If you are someone like me that likes trying so many treats and yummy recipes almost every day, the present regimen may not be easy in the long term. However, this diet is programmed to accommodate both long-term and short-term goals. There are three major diet plans to choose from to suit your desired eating habit.

The 5&1 plan may not be easy in the long-term, but there are over 60 fueling options to work with. Moreover, you have a plethora of resources where you can get recipes, including this cookbook with so many mouthwatering recipes to make.

Unlike most weight-loss diets, you don't need to stress yourself counting calories, points, or carbs. Though they are needed for reference purposes, you don't need to kill yourself over it as long as the meals you are taking are lean and green meals.

Interestingly, you can easily eat out while on this diet. The main thing is for you to understand the guidelines and follow them judiciously. You can as well download the eating out guide from the company website to help you easily navigate the buffets and eateries.

CHAPTER 1:

What to Eat

Best Foods for LEAN and GREEN Diet

Your homemade meals are expected to be mostly low-carb vegetables, lean proteins, and a few healthy fats. Low-carb beverages such as coffee, water, tea, unsweetened almond milk, etc, are allowed, but in small amounts.

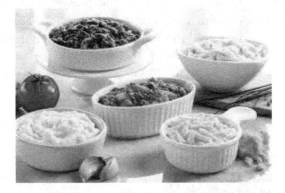

- The recommended foods for your lean and green meals are;

- Fish and Shellfish: trout, halibut, salmon, shrimp, tuna, crab, lobster, scallops.

- Meat: Lean beef, pork chop, tenderloin, turkey, chicken, lamb.

- Eggs: egg whites, whole eggs, and egg beaters.

- Soy: tofu

- Oil: vegetable oils - flaxseed, olive, canola, walnut, lemon oil, etc

- Fats: avocado, olives, almonds, pistachios, reduced-fat margarine, walnuts, etc.

- Vegetables: zucchini, cauliflower, celery, mushrooms, eggplant, pepper, spinach, cucumbers, squash, broccoli, collard, jicama, etc.

- Snacks (sugar-free): mints, popsicle, gum, gelatin, etc.

- Beverages (sugar-free): coffee, water, tea, almond milk, etc.

- Seasoning and condiments: spices, dried herbs, salsa, cocktail sauce, yellow mustard, lemon juice, soy sauce, lime juice, etc.

Avoid These Foods

Except for the carbs in the Fuelings, the present diet restricts most foods and beverages with carb content. Some fats are not allowed, including fried foods. Avoid the following foods in your daily meals;

- Refined grains: including pasta, flour tortillas, cookies, white rice, white bread, cakes, biscuits, etc.

- Whole fat dairy: including yogurt, milk, and cheese.

- Fried foods: including fish, veggies, meats, pastries, etc.

- Fats: like coconut oil, butter, etc.

- Alcohol: all types.

- Beverages: like an energy drink, fruit juice, sweet tea, soda, etc

If you are on the 5&1 plan, you need to avoid the following foods in your daily meal. You can introduce them in the transition phase;

- Starchy veggies: white potatoes, sweet potatoes, peas, and corn.

- Whole grains: brown rice, whole grain bread, whole-wheat pasta, etc.

- Low-fat dairy: cheese, yogurt, and milk.

- Legumes: beans, peas, soybeans, lentils, etc.

- Fruits: fresh fruits. Eat more berries when you enter the transition phase.

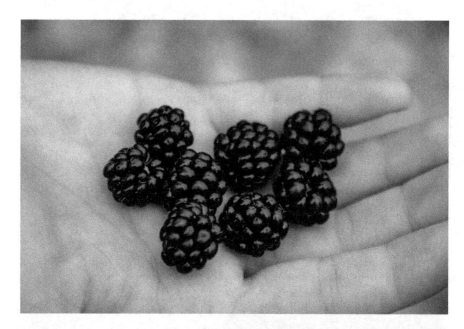

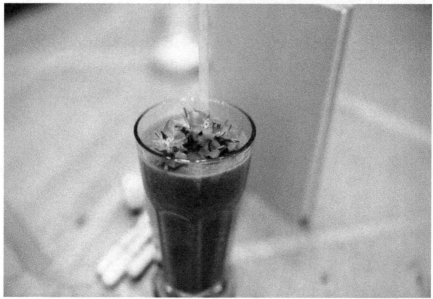

CHAPTER 2:

Lean and Green Recipes

1.   Quick Lemon Pepper Salmon

Preparation Time: 10 minutes

Cooking Time: 18 minutes

Servings: 2

Ingredients:

- 1 ½ lbs salmon fillets

- ½ tsp ground black pepper

- 1 tsp dried oregano

- 2 garlic cloves, minced

- ¼ cup olive oil

- 1 lemon juice

- 1 tsp sea salt

Directions:

1. In a large bowl, mix together lemon juice, olive oil, garlic, oregano, black pepper, and salt.

2. Add fish fillets in bowl and coat well with the marinade, and place in the refrigerator for 15 minutes.

3. Preheat the grill.

4. Brush grill grates with oil.

5. Place marinated salmon fillets on a hot grill and cook for 4 minutes, then turn salmon fillets to the other side and cook for 4 minutes more.

Nutrition: Calories 340, Fat 6, Carbs 31, Protein 28

2.   Tomatillo and Green Chili Pork Stew

Preparation Time: 10 minutes

Cooking Time: 20 minutes

Servings: 4

Ingredients:

- 2 scallions, chopped

- 2 cloves of garlic

- 1 lb. tomatillos, trimmed and chopped

- 2 serrano chilies, seeds, and membranes

- ½ tsp of dried Mexican oregano (or you can use regular oregano)

- 1 ½ lb. of boneless pork loin, to be cut into bite-sized cubes

- ¼ cup of cilantro, chopped

- ¼ tablespoon (each) salt and paper

- 1 jalapeno, seeds and membranes to be removed and thinly sliced

- 1 cup of sliced radishes

- 4 lime wedges

Directions:

1. Combine all ingredients and puree until smooth

2. Season with pepper & salt, and cover it simmers. Simmer on the heat for approximately 20 minutes.

Nutrition: Calories 356, Fat 19, Carbs 11, Protein 23

3.   Optavia Cloud Bread

Preparation Time: 25 minutes

Cooking Time: 35 minutes

Servings: 3

Ingredients:

- ½ cup of Fat-free 0% Plain Greek Yogurt (4.4 0z)

- 3 Eggs, Separated

- 16 teaspoon Cream of Tartar

- 1 Packet sweetener (a granulated sweetener just like stevia)

Directions:

1. For about 30 minutes before making this meal, place the

   Kitchen Aid Bowl and the whisk attachment in the freezer.

2. Preheat your oven to 30 degrees

3. Remove the mixing bowl and whisk attachment from the freezer

4. Separate the eggs. Now put the egg whites in the Kitchen Aid

   Bowl, and they should be in a different medium-sized bowl.

5. In the medium-sized bowl containing the yolks, mix in the

   sweetener and yogurt.

6. In the bowl containing the egg white, add in the cream of tartar.

   Beat this mixture until the egg whites turn to stiff peaks.

7. Now, take the egg yolk mixture and carefully fold it into the egg

   whites. Be cautious and avoid over-stirring.

8. Place baking paper on a baking tray and spray with cooking

   spray.

9. Scoop out 6 equally-sized "blobs" of the "dough" onto the parchment paper.

10. Bake for about 25-35 minutes (make sure you check when it is 25 minutes, in some ovens, they are done at this timestamp). You will know they are done as they will get brownish at the top and have some crack.

11. Most people like them cold against being warm

12. Most people like to re-heat in a toast oven or toaster to get them a little bit crispy.

13. Your serving size should be about 2 pieces.

Nutrition: Calories 234, Fat 4, Carbs 5, Protein 23

4. Avocado Lime Shrimp Salad

Preparation Time: 15 minutes

Cooking Time: 0 minutes

Servings: 2

Ingredients:

- 14 ounces of jumbo cooked shrimp, peeled and deveined; chopped

- 4 ½ ounces of avocado, diced

- 1 ½ cup of tomato, diced

- ¼ cup of chopped green onion

- ¼ cup of jalapeno with the seeds removed, diced fine

- 1 teaspoon of olive oil

- 2 tablespoons of lime juice

- 1/8 teaspoon of salt

- 1 tablespoon of chopped cilantro

Directions:

1. Get a small bowl and combine green onion, olive oil, lime juice, pepper, a pinch of salt. Wait for about 5 minutes for all of them to marinate and mellow the flavor of the onion.

2. Get a large bowl and combine chopped shrimp, tomato, avocado, jalapeno. Combine all of the ingredients, add cilantro, and gently toss.

3. Add pepper and salt as desired.

Nutrition: Calories 312, Fat 6, Carbs 15, Protein 26

CHAPTER 3:

Fuelings

5.   Blueberry Muffins

Preparation time: 35 minutes

Cooking time: 20 minutes

Servings: 12

Ingredients:

- 2 eggs

- 1/2 cup fresh blueberries

- 1 cup heavy cream

- 2 cups almond flour

- 1/4 tsp lemon zest

- 1/2 tsp lemon extract

- 1 tsp baking powder

- 5 drops stevia

- 1/4 cup butter, melted

Directions:

1. Preheat the oven to 350 F. Line muffin tin with cupcake liners and set aside.

2. Add eggs into the bowl and whisk until mix.

3. Add remaining ingredients and mix to combine.

4. Pour mixture into the prepared muffin tin and bake for 25 minutes.

5. Serve and enjoy.

Nutrition: calories 190, Fat 17, Carbs 5, Protein 5

6. Chia Pudding

Preparation time: 15 minutes

Cooking time: 20 minutes

Servings: 2

Ingredients:

- 4 tbsp chia seeds

- 1 cup unsweetened coconut milk

- 1/2 cup raspberries

Directions:

1. Add raspberry and coconut milk into a blender and blend until smooth.

2. Pour mixture into the glass jar.

3. Add chia seeds in a jar and stir well.

4. Seal the jar with a lid and shake well and place in the refrigerator

    for 3 hours.

5. Serve chilled and enjoy.

Nutrition: calories 360, Fat 33, Carbs 13, Protein 6

7.   Avocado Pudding

Preparation time: 10 minutes

Cooking time: 20 minutes

Servings: 10

Ingredients:

- 2 ripe avocados, peeled, pitted, and cut into pieces

- 1 tbsp fresh lime juice

- 14 oz can coconut milk

- 2 tsp liquid stevia

- 2 tsp vanilla

Directions:

1. Add all ingredients into the blender and blend until smooth.

2. Serve immediately and enjoy.

Nutrition: calories 317, Fat 30, Carbs 9, Protein 3

8. Peanut Butter Coconut Popsicle

Preparation time: 10 minutes **Cooking time:** 20 minutes

Servings: 10

Ingredients:

- 1/2 cup peanut butter

- 1 tsp liquid stevia

- 2 cans unsweetened coconut milk

Directions:

1. Add all ingredients into the blender and blend until smooth.

2. Pour mixture into the Popsicle molds and place in the freezer for 4 hours or until set.

3. Serve and enjoy.

CHAPTER 4:

Lunch Recipes

9.   Easy Low Carb Cauliflower Pizza Crust

Preparation time: 15 minutes

Cooking time: 8 minutes

Servings: 8

Ingredients:

- 3 cups almond flour

- 3 tbsp butter, then melted

- ⅓ tsp salt

- Cauliflower

- 3 large eggs

Directions

1. Preheat oven to 350°F. In a bowl, mix the almond flour, butter, salt, and eggs until a dough forms. Mold the dough into a ball and place it in between two wide parchment papers on a flat surface. Place the cauliflower on the dough.

2. Use a rolling pin to roll it out into a circle of a quarter-inch thickness. Place the cauliflower on the dough.

3. Slide the pizza dough into the pizza pan and remove the parchment papers. Bake the dough for 20 minutes.

Nutrition: Calories 234, Fat 16, Carbs 8, Protein 12

10.　Fresh Tomato Basil Soup

Preparation time: 15 minutes

Cooking time: 40 minutes

Servings: 4

Ingredients:

- ¼ c. olive oil

- ½ c. heavy cream

- 1 lb. tomatoes, fresh 4 c. chicken broth, divided

- 4 cloves garlic, fresh Sea salt & pepper to taste

Directions:

1. Preheat oven to 400° Fahrenheit and line a baking sheet with foil.

2. Remove the cores from your tomatoes and place them on the baking sheet along with the cloves of garlic.

3. Drizzle tomatoes and garlic with olive oil, salt, and pepper.

4. Roast for 30 minutes.

5. Pull the tomatoes out of the oven and place them into a blender, along with the juices that have dripped onto the pan during roasting.

6. Add two cups of the chicken broth to the blender.

7. Blend until smooth, then strain the mixture into a large saucepan or a pot.

8. While the pan is on the stove, whisk the remaining two cups of broth and the cream into the soup.

9. Simmer for about ten minutes.

10. Season to taste, then serve hot!

Nutrition: Calories 255, Fat 20, Carbs 6, Protein 7

11.   Creamy Beef Stroganoff

Preparation time: 10 minutes

Cooking time: 20 minutes

Servings: 4

Ingredients:

- 1 lb beef strips

- 3/4 cup mushrooms, sliced

- 1 small onion, chopped

- 1 tbsp butter

- 2 tbsp olive oil

- 2 tbsp green onion, chopped

- 1/4 cup sour cream

- 1 cup chicken broth

- Pepper

- Salt

Directions:

1. Add meat in bowl and coat with 1 teaspoon oil, pepper, and salt.

2. Heat remaining oil in a pan.

3. Add meat to the pan and cook until golden brown on both sides.

4. Transfer meat to a bowl and set aside.

5. Add butter to the same pan.

6. Add onion and cook until onion softened.

7. Add mushrooms and sauté until the liquid is absorbed.

8. Add broth and cook until the sauce thickened.

9. Add sour cream, green onion, and meat and stir well.

10. Cook over medium-high heat for 3-4 minutes.

11. Serve and enjoy.

Nutrition: Calories 345, Fat 20, Carbs 3, Protein 35

12.　Pork Bowls

Preparation time: 15 minutes

Cooking time: 15 minutes

Servings: 4

Ingredients:

- 1¼ pounds pork belly, cut into bite-size pieces

- 2 Tbsp tamari soy sauce

- 1 Tbsp rice vinegar

- 2 cloves garlic, smashed

- 3 oz butter

- 1 pound Brussels sprouts, rinsed, trimmed, halved, or quartered

- ½ leek, chopped

- Salt and ground black pepper to taste

Directions:

1. Fry the pork over medium-high heat until it is starting to turn golden brown.

2. Combine the garlic cloves, butter, and brussel sprouts. Add to the pan, whisk well and cook until the sprouts turn golden brown.

3. Stir the soy sauce and rice vinegar together and pour the sauce into the pan.

4. Sprinkle with salt and pepper. Top with chopped leek.

Nutrition: Calories 421, Fat 22, Carbs 7, Protein 19

CHAPTER 5:

Dinner Recipes

13.   Dill Relish on White Sea Bass

Preparation Time: 10 minutes

Cooking Time: 12 minutes

Servings: 4

Ingredients:

1 ½ tablespoon chopped white onion

1 ½ teaspoon chopped fresh dill

1 lemon, quartered

1 teaspoon Dijon mustard

1 teaspoon lemon juice

1 teaspoon pickled baby capers, drained

4 pieces of 4-oz white sea bass fillets

Directions:

Preheat oven to 375oF.

Mix lemon juice, mustard, dill, capers and onions in a small bowl.

Prepare four aluminum foil squares and place 1 fillet per foil.

Squeeze a lemon wedge per fish.

Evenly divide into 4 the dill spread and drizzle over fillet.

Close the foil over the fish securely and pop in the oven.

Bake for 12 minutes or until fish is cooked through.

Remove from foil and transfer to a serving platter, serve and enjoy.

Nutrition:

Calories: 115

Protein: 7g

Fat: 1g

Carbs: 12g

14.   Quinoa With Vegetables

Preparation Time: 10 minutes

Cooking Time: 5 to 6 hours

Servings: 8

Ingredients:

2 cups quinoa, rinsed and drained

2 onions, chopped 2 carrots, peeled and sliced

1 cup sliced cremini mushrooms 3 garlic cloves, minced

4 cups low-sodium vegetable broth

1/2 teaspoon salt

1 teaspoon dried marjoram leaves

1/8 teaspoon freshly ground black pepper

Directions:

In a 6-quart slow cooker, mix all of the ingredients.

Cover and cook on low for 5 to 6 hours, or until the quinoa and

vegetables are tender.

Stir the mixture and serve.

Nutrition:

Calories: 204 Cal

Carbohydrates: 35 g

Sugar: 4 g Fiber: 4 g

Fat: 3 g Saturated Fat: 0 g

Protein: 7 g Sodium: 229 mg

15. Chicken Goulash

Preparation Time: 10 minutes

Cooking Time: 17 minutes

Servings: 6

Ingredients:

4 oz. chive stems

2 green peppers, chopped

1 teaspoon olive oil

14 oz. ground chicken

2 tomatoes

½ cup chicken stock

2 garlic cloves, sliced

1 teaspoon salt

1 teaspoon ground black pepper

1 teaspoon mustard

Directions:

Chop chives roughly.

Spray the air fryer basket tray with the olive oil.

Preheat the air fryer to 365 F.

Put the chopped chives in the air fryer basket tray.

Add the chopped green pepper and cook the vegetables for 5 minutes.

Add the ground chicken.

Chop the tomatoes into the small cubes and add them in the air fryer mixture too.

Cook the mixture for 6 minutes more.

Add the chicken stock, sliced garlic cloves, salt, ground black pepper, and mustard.

Mix well to combine.

Cook the goulash for 6 minutes more.

Nutrition:

Calories: 161

Fat: 6.1g

Carbs: 6g

Protein: 20.3g

16.   Chicken & Turkey Meatloaf

Preparation Time: 15 minutes

Cooking Time: 25 minutes

Servings: 12

Ingredients:

3 tablespoon butter

10 oz. ground turkey

7 oz. ground chicken

1 teaspoon dried dill

½ teaspoon ground coriander

2 tablespoons almond flour

1 tablespoon minced garlic

3 oz. fresh spinach

1 teaspoon salt

1 egg

½ tablespoon paprika

1 teaspoon sesame oil

Directions:

Put the ground turkey and ground chicken in a large bowl.

Sprinkle the meat with dried dill, ground coriander, almond flour, minced garlic, salt, and paprika.

Then chop the fresh spinach and add it to the ground poultry mixture.

break the egg into the meat mixture and mix well until you get a smooth texture.

Great the air fryer basket tray with the olive oil.

Preheat the air fryer to 350 F.

Roll the ground meat mixture gently to make the flat layer.

Put the butter in the center of the meat layer.

Make the shape of the meatloaf from the ground meat mixture. Use your fingertips for this step.

Place the meatloaf in the air fryer basket tray.

Cook for 25 minutes.

When the meatloaf is cooked allow it to rest before serving.

Nutrition:

Calories: 142 Fat: 9.8 g Carbs: 1.7g

Protein: 13g

17.　　Turkey Meatballs with Dried Dill

Preparation Time: 15 minutes

Cooking Time: 11 minutes

Servings: 9

Ingredients:

1-pound ground turkey

1 teaspoon chili flakes

¼ cup chicken stock

2 tablespoon dried dill

1 egg

1 teaspoon salt

1 teaspoon paprika

1 tablespoon coconut flour

2 tablespoons heavy cream

1 teaspoon olive oil

Directions:

in a bowl, whisk the egg with a fork.

Add the ground turkey and chili flakes.

Sprinkle the mixture with dried dill, salt, paprika, coconut flour, and mix

it up.

Make the meatballs from the ground turkey mixture.

Preheat the air fryer to 360 F.

Grease the air fryer basket tray with the olive oil.

Then put the meatballs inside.

Cook the meatballs for 6 minutes – for 3 minutes on each side.

Sprinkle the meatballs with the heavy cream.

Cook the meatballs for 5 minutes more.

When the turkey meatballs are cooked – let them rest for 2-3 minutes.

Nutrition:

Calories: 124 Fat: 7.9g Carbs: 1.2g

Protein: 14.8g

CHAPTER 6:

Soup and Salads

18.   Alkaline Pumpkin Tomato Soup

Preparation Time: 15 minutes

Cooking Time: 30 minutes

Servings: 3-4

Ingredients:

- 1 quart of water (if accessible: soluble water)

- 400g new tomatoes, stripped and diced

- 1 medium-sized sweet pumpkin

- 5 yellow onions

- 1 tbsp. cold squeezed additional virgin olive oil

- 2 tsp. ocean salt or natural salt

- Touch of cayenne pepper

- Your preferred spices (discretionary)

- Bunch of new parsley

Directions:

1. Cut onions in little pieces and sauté with some oil in a significant pot.

2. Cut the pumpkin down the middle, at that point remove the stem and scoop out the seeds.

3. Finally, scoop out the fragile living creature and put it in the pot.

4. Include the tomatoes and the water and cook for around 20 minutes.

5. At that point, empty the soup into a food processor and blend well for a couple of moments. Sprinkle with salt, pepper, and other spices.

6. Fill bowls and trimming with new parsley. Make the most of your alkalizing soup!

Nutrition: calories 190, fat 3, carbs 18, protein 11

19. Alkaline Pumpkin Coconut Soup

Preparation Time: 10 minutes

Cooking Time: 15 minutes

Servings: 3-4

Ingredients:

- 2lb pumpkin

- 6 cups of water (best: soluble water delivered with a water ionizer)

- 1 cup low-fat coconut milk

- 5 ounces of potatoes

- 2 major onions

- 3 ounces leek

- 1 bunch of new parsley

- 1 touch of nutmeg

- 1 touch of cayenne pepper

- 1 tsp. ocean salt or natural salt

- 4 tbsp. cold squeezed additional virgin olive oil

Directions:

1. As a matter of first significance: cut the onions, the pumpkin, and the potatoes just as the hole into little pieces.

2. At that point, heat the olive oil in a significant pot and sauté the onions for a couple of moments.

3. At that point, include the water and heat up the pumpkin, potatoes, and the leek until delicate.

4. Include coconut milk.

5. Presently utilize a hand blender and puree for around 1 moment. The soup should turn out to be extremely velvety.

6. Season with salt, pepper, and nutmeg. Lastly, include the parsley and appreciate this alkalizing pumpkin soup hot or cold!

Nutrition: calories 90, fat 3, carbs 23, protein 1

20.   Cold Cauliflower-Coconut Soup

Preparation Time: 7 minutes

Cooking Time: 20 minutes

Servings: 3-4

Ingredients:

- 1 pound (450g) new cauliflower

- 1 ¼ cup (300ml) unsweetened coconut milk

- 1 cup of water (best: antacid water)

- 2 tbsp. new lime juice

- 1/3 cup cold squeezed additional virgin olive oil

- 1 cup new coriander leaves, slashed

- Spot of salt and cayenne pepper

- 1 bunch of unsweetened coconut chips

Directions:

1. Steam cauliflower for around 10 minutes.

2. At that point, set up the cauliflower with coconut milk and water in a food processor and get it started until extremely smooth.

3. Include new lime squeeze, salt and pepper, a large portion of the cleaved coriander, and the oil and blend for an additional couple of moments.

4. Pour in soup bowls and embellishment with coriander and coconut chips. Appreciate!

Nutrition: calories 190, fat 1, carbs 21, protein 6

CHAPTER 7:

Smoothie Recipes

21.   Apple Spinach Cucumber Smoothie

Preparation Time: 10 minutes

Cooking Time: 0 minutes

Servings: 1

Ingredients:

- 3/4 cup water

- 1/2 green apple, diced

- 3/4 cup spinach

- 1/2 cucumber

Directions:

1. Add all ingredients to the blender and blend until smooth and

   creamy.

2. Serve immediately and enjoy.

Nutrition: calories 90, fat 1, carbs 21, protein 1

22.   Refreshing Lime Smoothie

Preparation Time: 10 minutes

Cooking Time: 0 minutes

Servings: 2

Ingredients:

- 1 cup ice cubes

- 20 drops liquid stevia

- 2 fresh lime, peeled and halved

- 1 tablespoon lime zest, grated

- 1/2 cucumber, chopped

- 1 avocado, pitted and peeled

- 2 cups spinach

- 1 tablespoon creamed coconut

- 3/4 cup coconut water

Directions:

1. Add all ingredients to the blender and blend until smooth and

   creamy.

2. Serve immediately and enjoy.

Nutrition: calories 312, fat 3, carbs 28, protein 4

23.   Broccoli Green Smoothie

Preparation Time: 10 minutes

Cooking Time: 0 minutes

Servings: 2

Ingredients:

- 1 celery, peeled and chopped

- 1 lemon, peeled

- 1 apple, diced 1 banana

- 1 cup spinach 1/2 cup broccoli

Directions:

1. Add all ingredients to the blender and blend until smooth and

   creamy.

2. Serve immediately and enjoy.

Nutrition: calories 121, fat 1, carbs 18, protein 1

CHAPTER 8:

Fish and Seafood Recipes

24.   **Mango** Tilapia **Fillets**

Preparation Time: 10 minutes

Cooking Time: 15 minutes

Servings: 4

Ingredients:

- ¼ cup coconut flakes

- 5 oz mango, peeled

- 1/3 cup shallot, chopped

- 1 teaspoon ground turmeric

- 1 cup of water

- 1 bay leaf

- 12 oz tilapia fillets

- 1 chili pepper, chopped

- 1 tablespoon coconut oil

- ½ teaspoon salt

- 1 teaspoon paprika

Directions:

1. Blend together coconut flakes, mango, shallot, ground turmeric, and water.

2. After this, melt coconut oil in the saucepan.

3. Sprinkle the tilapia fillets with salt and paprika.

4. Then place them in the hot coconut oil and roast for 1 minute from each side.

5. Add chili pepper, bay leaf, and blended mango mixture.

6. Close the lid and cook the fish for 10 minutes over medium heat.

Nutrition: calories 342, fat 1, carbs 18, protein 23

25.   **Lemon** Butter **Fillet**

Preparation Time: 20 minutes

Cooking Time: 30 minutes

Servings: 5

Ingredients:

- 1/2 cup butter

- 1 lemon, juiced

- 1 teaspoon ground black pepper

- 1/2 teaspoon dried basil

- 3 cloves garlic, minced

- 6 (4 ounce) fillets cod

- 2 tablespoons lemon pepper

Directions:

1. Preheat oven to 350 degrees F.

2. Melt the butter in a medium saucepan over medium heat. Bring to a boil.

3. Arrange cod fillets in a single layer on a medium baking sheet. Cover with 1/2 the butter mixture, and sprinkle with lemon pepper. Cover with foil.

Nutrition: calories 169, fat 4, carbs 5, protein 33

26. Fish Soup

Preparation Time: 10 minutes

Cooking Time: 30 minutes

Servings: 5

Ingredients:

- 1/2 onion, chopped

- 1 clove garlic, minced

- 1 tablespoon chili powder

- 1 1/2 cups chicken broth

- 1 teaspoon ground cumin

- 1/2 cup chopped green bell pepper

- 1/2 cup shrimp

- 1/2 pound cod fillets

- 3/4 cup plain yogurt

Directions:

1. Spray a large saucepan with the cooking spray over medium-high heat. Add the onions and sauté, stirring often, for about 5 minutes. Add the garlic and chili powder and sauté for 2 more minutes.

2. Then add the chicken broth and cumin, stirring well. Bring to a boil, reduce heat to low, cover and simmer for 20 minutes.

3. Next, add green bell pepper, shrimp, and cod. Return to a boil, then reduce heat to low, cover, and simmer for another 5 minutes. Gradually stir in the yogurt until heated through.

Nutrition: calories 390, fat 5, carbs 28, protein 41

27. Cod Egg Sandwich

Preparation Time: 10 minutes

Cooking Time: 10 minutes

Servings: 2

Ingredients:

- 2 (5 ounce) can cod, drained 6 hard-cooked eggs, peeled and chopped

- 2 cups chopped celery 2 tablespoons mayonnaise

- Pepper to taste 8 slices white bread

Directions:

1. In a medium bowl, stir together the cod, eggs, celery, and mayonnaise. Season with pepper to taste. Place half of the

mixture onto 1 slice of bread and the other half on another slice

of bread. Top with remaining slices of bread. Serve.

Nutrition: calories 110, fat 16, carbs 18, protein 43

28. Tuna Mushroom Casserole

Preparation Time: 10 minutes

Cooking Time: 53 minutes

Servings: 3

Ingredients:

- 2 cups macaroni

- 2 (5 ounce) cans tuna, drained

- 1 (10 ounce) can mushrooms, drained

- 1 cup water

- 1 1/3 cups soy milk

- 1/4 teaspoon freshly ground black pepper

- 1 cup dry white bread crumbs

- 3 tablespoons melted butter

- 2 teaspoons dried thyme, crushed

Directions:

1. In a mixing bowl, combine bread crumbs, butter, and thyme. Mix well. Sprinkle over the top of the tuna mixture.

2. Bake uncovered in a preheated oven until bubbling and golden brown, about 40 minutes.

Nutrition: calories 422, fat 12, carbs 18, protein 1

29.   Ginger and Lime Salmon

Preparation Time: 15 minutes

Cooking Time: 15 minutes

Servings: 2

Ingredients:

- 1 (1 1/2-pound) salmon fillet

- 1 tablespoon olive oil

- 1 teaspoon oregano

- 1 teaspoon ground black pepper

- 1 (1 inch) piece fresh ginger root, peeled and thinly sliced

- 6 cloves garlic, minced

- 1 lime, thinly sliced

Directions:

1. Season with oregano and black pepper.

2. Broil salmon until hot and beginning to turn opaque, about 10 minutes; watch carefully.

3. If the broiler has a High setting, turn the broiler to that setting and continue broiling until salmon is cooked through and flakes easily with a fork, 5 to 10 more minutes.

Nutrition: calories 121, fat 32, carbs 18, protein 43

30. Lemon Rosemary Salmon with Garlic

Preparation Time: 15 minutes **Cooking Time:** 35 minutes

Servings: 3

Ingredients:

- 1/4 cup butter, melted 1/4 cup white wine

- 1 lemon, juiced 5 cloves garlic, chopped

- 1 bunch fresh rosemary, stems trimmed 1 (1 pound) salmon

  fillet

Directions:

1. Preheat oven to 375 degrees F. Mix butter, white wine, lemon

   juice, and garlic together in a small bowl. Bake for 25 minutes.

Nutrition: calories 324, fat 12, carbs 1, protein 41

CHAPTER 9:

Poultry Recipes

31.   Baked Chicken Breasts

Preparation Time: 13 minutes

Cooking Time: 20 minutes

Servings: 6

Ingredients:

- 6 chicken breasts, skinless & boneless

- 1/4 tsp. paprika

- 1/2 tsp. garlic salt

- 1 tsp. Italian seasoning

- 2 tbsp. olive oil

- 1/4 tsp. pepper

Directions:

1. Insert wire rack in rack position 6. Select bake, set temperature 390 F, timer for 25 minutes. Press start to preheat the oven.

2. Brush chicken with oil. Mix together Italian seasoning, garlic salt, paprika, and pepper and rub all over the chicken.

3. Arrange chicken breasts on a roasting pan and bake for 25 minutes or until internal temperature reaches 165 F.

4. Slice and serve. **Nutrition:** Calories 321, Fat 15, Carbs 1, Protein 42

32.   Flavors Balsamic Chicken

Preparation Time: 12 minutes

Cooking Time: 25 minutes

Servings: 4

Ingredients:

- 4 chicken breasts, skinless and boneless

- 2 tsp. dried oregano

- 2 garlic cloves, minced

- 1/2 cup balsamic vinegar

- 2 tbsp. soy sauce

- 1/4 cup of oil

- Pepper

- Salt

Directions:

1. Insert wire rack in rack position 6. Select bake, set temperature 390 F, timer for 25 minutes. Press start to preheat the oven.

2. In a bowl, mix together soy sauce, oil, black pepper, oregano, garlic, and vinegar.

3. Place chicken in a baking dish and pour soy sauce mixture over chicken. Let it sit for 10 minutes. Bake chicken for 25 minutes. Serve and enjoy.

Nutrition: Calories 401, Fat 23, Carbs 2, Protein 42

33. Simple & Delicious Chicken Thighs

Preparation Time: 10 minutes

Cooking Time: 35 minutes

Servings: 6

Ingredients:

- 6 chicken thighs

- 2 tsp. poultry seasoning

- 2 tbsp. oil

- Pepper Salt

Directions:

1. Insert wire rack in rack position 6. Select bake, set temperature 390 F, timer for 40 minutes. Press start to preheat the oven.

2. Brush chicken with oil and rub with poultry seasoning, pepper, and salt.

3. Arrange chicken on roasting pan and bake for 35-40 minutes or until internal temperature reaches 165 F.

4. Serve and enjoy.

Nutrition: Calories 319, Fat 15, Carbs 1, Protein 42

34. Perfect Baked Chicken Breasts

Preparation Time: 10 minutes

Cooking Time: 30 minutes

Servings: 4

Ingredients:

- 4 chicken breasts, bone-in & skin-on

- 1 tsp. oil (Olive)

- 1/4 tsp. black pepper

- 1/2 tsp. kosher salt

Directions:

1. Insert wire rack in rack position 6. Select bake, set temperature 375 F, timer for 30 minutes. Press start to preheat the oven.

2. Brush chicken with oil and season with salt

3. Place chicken on roasting pan and bake for 30 minutes.

4. Serve and enjoy.

Nutrition: Calories 288, Fat 12, Carbs 1, Protein 42

CHAPTER 10:

Vegan & Vegetarian

35.   Buffalo Cauliflower – Onion Dip

Preparation time:

Cooking Time:

Servings: 2

Ingredients:

- ¾ head of Cauliflower

- ¾ cup of Buffalo sauce

- Seasoning and spice: Garlic powder (1½ tsp.) and salt (to taste)

- Creamy dipping sauce: French onion dip (or any sauce of your choice)

- Celery

- 3 tbsp. Olive oil

Directions:

1. Cut the head of cauliflower into tiny florets into a big bowl.

2. Add and mix the cauliflower with the buffalo sauce and the rest of the ingredients apart from the dip sauce and celery sticks.

3. Grease the air fryer rack lightly. Preheat the air fryer to 375°F.

4. Transfer the well-mixed cauliflower to the air fryer in batches if they cannot all fit into the rack.

5. Set the timer to 10-12 minutes and cook until the cauliflower florets are tender and browned a bit.

6. Serve warm with the celery sticks and dipping sauce of your choice. In my own case, french onion dip.

Nutrition: Calories 200, Fat 4, Carbs 190, Protein 9.

36.   Baked Apple

Preparation time: 15 minutes

Cooking Time: 25 minutes

Servings: 2

Ingredients:

- 2 Apples

- Oats (as a topping)

- 3 tsp. melted margarine/butter

- ½ tsp. Cinnamon

- ½ tsp. nutmeg powder

- 4 Tbsp. raisins

- ½ cup of water

Directions:

1. Wash and dry apples.

2. Cut the apples in half and use a spoon or knife to cut out some of the flesh.

3. Add the melted margarine, cinnamon, nutmeg powder, chopped raisins, and oats into a small bowl and mix.

4. Preheat the air fryer to 350°F.

5. Place the apples into the drip pan at the bottom of the air fryer.

6. Put the mixture into the center of the apples using a spoon.

7. Pour water into the pan.

8. Set the timer to 15-20 minutes for it to bake till apples are tender and fillings are crisp and browned.

9. Cover the fillings with foil if they seem to be browning quickly.

10. Serve warm and enjoy.

Nutrition: Calories 380, Fat 6, Carbs 170, Protein 14.

37.   Eggplant Parmesan

Preparation time: 20 minutes

Cooking Time: 20 minutes

Servings: 3

Ingredients:

- 2 Eggplants

- 1 cup Whole wheat bread crumbs

- 1 cup Flour

- 1 cup Almond milk

- 4 tbsp. Vegan parmesan

- Spices: onion powder, pepper, garlic powder, and salt (to taste)

- Sauce: marinara

- Toppings: 1 cup mozzarella shreds

Directions:

1. Wash and dry eggplants.

2. Cut into slices.

3. Sieve flour to remove air bubbles into a bowl.

4. Mix whole wheat bread crumbs with vegan parmesan, onion powder, pepper, garlic powder, and salt together into a bowl.

5. Take the slices and dip into flour to be coated, then into the almond milk, and lastly into the mixture of vegan parmesan and spices.

6. Preheat the air fryer at 375°F.

7. Place eggplant slices into the air fryer rack.

8. Set the timer to 15-20 minutes, pressing the "Rotate" so that you can turn the slices halfway through.

9. Once golden brown on both sides, top with marinara and the mozzarella shreds and air fry for about 1-2 minutes to melt.

10. Serve warm and enjoy with pasta or any meal of your choice.

Nutrition: Calories 308, Fat 4, Carbs 54, Protein 8.

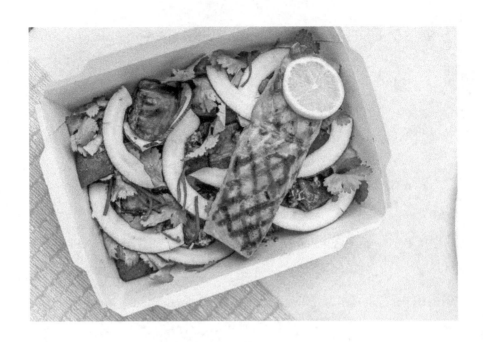

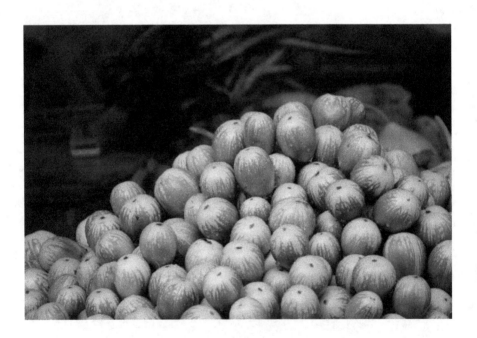

CHAPTER 11:

Pork recipes

38.　　Roasted Pepper Pork Prosciutto

Preparation Time: 20 minutes

Cooking Time: 60 minutes

Servings: 8

Ingredients

- 24 oz. pork cutlets

- Olive oil spray

- 12 oz. slices thin prosciutto

- 4 slices mozzarella

- 22 oz. roasted peppers

- 1 lemon

- 24 Spinach leaves

- 1 tbsp. olive oil

- 1/2 cup GF breadcrumbs

- Salt and fresh pepper

Directions

1. First, wash and dry the pork cutlets very well with paper towels. Add breadcrumbs to a bowl and in another second bowl, stir the olive oil, lemon juice, and pepper. Preheat the air fryer

toaster oven to 450°F. Slightly spray a baking dish with olive oil spray. Put each cutlet on a work surface such as a cutting board and lay 1/2 slice prosciutto, 1/2 slice cheese, 1 piece of roasted pepper, and 3 spinach leaves on one side of the pork cutlet. Roll it and put the seam side down on a dish. Dip down the pork in the olive oil and lemon juice after that into the breadcrumbs. Do the same with the pork left. Bake it for 25 to 30 minutes or until your desired crispness.

Nutrition: Calories: 268, Fat: 16g, Protein: 24g, Carbs: 7g, Fiber: 1g

CHAPTER 12:

Snack Recipes

39.   Cauliflower Spread

Preparation time: *10 minutes*

Cooking time: *7 hours*

Servings: *2*

Ingredients:

- 1 cup cauliflower florets

- 1 tablespoon mayonnaise

- ½ cup heavy cream

- 1 tablespoon lemon juice

- ½ teaspoon garlic powder

- ¼ teaspoon smoked paprika

- ¼ teaspoon mustard powder

- A pinch of salt and black pepper

Directions:

1. In your slow cooker, combine the cauliflower with the cream, mayonnaise, and the other ingredients, toss, put the lid on and cook on Low for 7 hours.

2. Transfer to a blender, pulse well, into bowls, and serve as a spread.

CHAPTER 13:

Appetizer Recipes

40.   Kale & Mushroom Frittata

Preparation Time: 15 minutes

Cooking Time: 30 minutes

Servings: 5

Ingredients:

- 8 eggs

- ½ cup unsweetened almond milk

- Salt and ground black pepper to taste

- 1 tablespoon olive oil

- 1 onion, chopped

- 1 garlic clove, minced

- 1 cup fresh mushrooms, chopped

- 1½ cups fresh kale, tough ribs removed and chopped

Directions:

1. Preheat oven to 350°F.

2. In a large bowl, place the eggs, coconut milk, salt, and black pepper, and beat well. Set aside.

3. In a large ovenproof wok, heat the oil over medium heat and sauté the onion and garlic for about 3–4 minutes.

4. Add the squash, kale, bell pepper, salt, and black pepper, and cook for about 8–10 minutes.

5. Stir in the mushrooms and cook for about 3–4 minutes.

6. Add the kale and cook for about 5 minutes.

7. Place the egg mixture on top evenly and cook for about 4 minutes, without stirring.

8. Transfer the wok to the oven and bake for about 12–15 minutes or until desired doneness.

9. Remove from the oven and place the frittata side for about 3–5 minutes before serving. Cut into desired sized wedges and serve.

Nutrition: calories 356, fat 2, carbs 4, protein 8

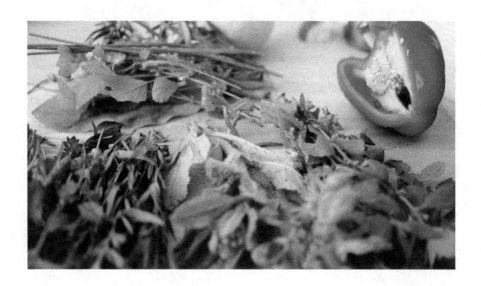

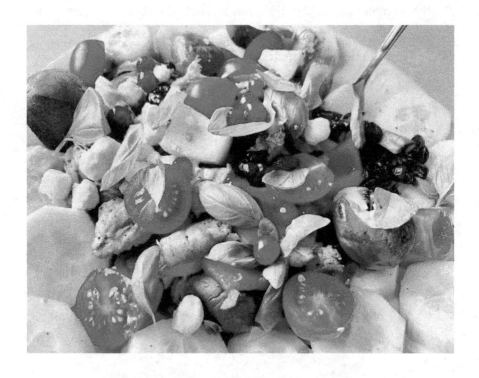

Conclusion

When you desire a structure and need to rapidly lose weight, the present diet is the perfect solution.

Its extremely low calories eating plans of the optavia diet will definitely help you to shed more pounds

Before you start any meal replacement diet plan, carefully consider if truly it possible for you to continue with a specific diet plan

When you have decided to stick with this regimen and make progress with your weight loss goal, ensure you have a brilliant knowledge about optimal health management to enable and archive the desired result effortlessly in the shortest period of time.

CPSIA information can be obtained
at www.ICGtesting.com
Printed in the USA
BVHW092303140621
609528BV00010B/1518